My Goliath
My journey with cancer
and
Chemotherapy treatments

My Goliath

Adrian Hamilton

Published by Adrian Hamilton, 2024.

MY GOLIATH

First edition. August 21, 2024.

Copyright © 2024 Adrian Hamilton.

ISBN: 979-8227393258

Written by Adrian Hamilton.

Adrian Hamilton

Dedication

This book is dedicated to those who had cancer and has conquered this disease I salute you, for those who are going through it along with the treatment, be patient it's a road you must travel. Pray to God and let him do the healing.

Acknowledgement

Thanks to the doctor who attended to me while going through the many tests, and finding what the symptoms I had was. Her dedication to her patients and her team of nurses working alongside her at St. Joseph Hospital in Hamilton. My thanks to the doctor and nurses at the Juravinski Cancer Hospital.

It was not a word you heard much while growing up, but knew of someone that had this incurable disease in the sixties called cancer. At that time they were no cure or medicine to be found, or available, and the word chemotherapy was not even thought of, as an alternative, for curing this deadly disease.

In fact, anyone with this disease were sent home to die depending on how severe and aggressive it was. You are luck if the doctor say you have a couple months at least, but if its a couple weeks imagine the arrangements that you have to make.

This disease was not as prevalent as today, but it was not something you broadcast. Growing up I never thought it would ever come my way, cause it was never in the foreground of my though, due to the many activities as a teenager. My activities took me into the forest eating anything I thought was good.

I ate lots of fruits, bananas, pineapples and drank lots of coconut water, smoking was never part of my activities. I ate new foods from my friends mother when she cooked, and whenever we went hunting or fishing.

Fast forward thirty years, living in a foreign country with a family, and not even giving the diseased called cancer anymore thought. I was always walking, riding and eating healthy, not even entertaining the thought of falling prey to any deadly disease.

Here I am, now living in this big country, where everything was advanced. I was always regular when it came to doing my daily routine, which i dubbed the three eases, for years upon end until one day on a Friday morning in August of 2005.

I woke up that morning with a constant pain deep within my collar bone area. It was such a persistent pain and tried alleviating the pain by drinking ginger tea,Canada dry ginger ale, cloves, orange peel and ginger tea, but none of these remedies helped.

The pain was beginning to get really unbearable, and could not stand it any longer. I walked to the hospital which was about a mike away, after arriving at the hospital around 3:00 p.m. went directly to the emergency department and registered as a patient. The nurse at the triage led me to a bed, and drew the curtain around me, and continued I continued waiting to be attended.

I remained in the cubicle with the curtains drawn around me for five hours. It was not until the hospital gown was being taken off, and said good-bye the nurse send someonr to look after me.

I could not understand why it took them five hours before coming to my aid. After looking after me i was sent home, and promise that someone would call me to follow up my case, and may want to do a couple test making sure that the cause of my pain was not serious.

Little did I know that this pain will cause me to go through so much. I eventually got a call from the doctor next morning around 8:00 am asking if its possible to get to the hospital by 9:3 a.m and my reply was yes, she said, go directly to the ultrasound department at the nurses station. They will be expecting you at that time, thanks was my reply, and hung up the phone.

After having a shower, got dressed and walked to the hospital, went directly to the ultrasound department and got registered. My test began within ten minutes after being registered. They began the test on my abdomen, no other place, but in one particular spot.

They did the test for at least twenty minutes, after testing was completed, dressed and came home. It was the week end and Just relaxed not knowing whet the doctor would be looking for, since my pain was in my shoulder area.

On Monday morning I received a call, to have another test done again at the same department at the hospital, and was not sure what was seen on the previous test to warrant another one, but it was the doctors order and it had to be done.

A day after the second test the doctor wanted two more tests done. This time it was another ultrasound and a barium enema, because she saw something on my colon and wanted to make sure it was nothing to worry about that she think was cancerous.

The tests had to be done today it being Wednesday around 1:00pm. I got to the ultrasound department once again on time as always, the ultrasound test was completed, and was taken to another room to have the barium enema test.

This is where a tube is put up your anus, and a white powder is released, making sure they were satisfied all the powder was completely finished. As you laid on your back another machine took pictures of your entire stomach.

It was not ba pleasant picture by any means. My next move was they had me sitting on the toilet waiting for me to expel the powder(in other words fart or pass gas) out of my system, which I did after twenty minutes of sitting on the toilet.

After it was all over I was told to go home. And the doctor will call you in a couple days if more tests are needed. It was exactly three dys later the doctor called, and said she wanted another test done, but will let me know the day and time.

It was now Friday morning the doctor called, and told me that I have to do a colonoscopy test, because the results of the ultrasound and barium enema tests were not conclusive. The fear of doing this test was now on my mind, with the what if's questions.

I was not aware what a colonoscopy test was, and it was explained to me in great detail, with the medication that have to be taken before the procedure can be carried out to have a good outcome.

After taking the medication that the doctor prescribed I had to make sure that any food or increment left in my stomach and bowel was depleted, for the procedure to be carried out without any complications. I could not eat anything the morning of the procedure, but was allowed a little sip of water.

The morning of my colonoscopy procedure I was driven to the hospital, proceeded to the oncology department, registered, and got dressed in a gown, stark naked with my butt showing. I had to lay on the bed and after all the necessary preparations were completed, it was my time to be wheeled into the area where the colonoscopy was to be performed.

The doctor that was doing the colonoscopy procedure introduced herself. And her team of nurses, explained what she was going to do. I was given an anesthetic injection and shortly after before, I could finishing counting from ten backwards, was fast asleep.

I woke up in the recovery room, not knowing what happened or took place. After being given the okay to go home after recovering although still wobbly walking my ride to the entrance door was in a wheelchair, and then driven home.

I was very hungry after the colonoscopy and had something light to eat, because what I had gone through this morning, and did not want to eat anything heavy. The day found me sleeping and woke up after six hours still feeling the effects which passed a couple hours.

My expectation was that the doctor was going to call me the same day with the results but it was not, and I was not waiting around for a call. I had errands to do and it was also my way of not thinking about the outcome of my colonoscopy, and what the doctors finding was and what it would mean for me.

Three days after the colonoscopy procedure the doctor's office called me. She said that it was imperative to see her the next day at her office at the hospital at 9:00 am, all I coils think of at that time was, is it good or bad news?

This kept me worried, and all I could hope for then, that it was good news and there was nothing to worry about. At the appointed time we drove to the doctors office at the hospital. We knocked on her door, and she said come in have a seat.

She looked at me called me by my name and said, a byopsy was done during the colonoscopy procedure, and found polyps that was cancerous, and yes you do have cancer of the colon.

It has not spread but you need to be operated on soon as possible, to be truthful within a week. The good news is it was caught early had it not harm could have been done and spreading of the cancerous polyps cause damage.

Doctor what are my chance of it not returning was my question? Your chance of it not returning is very good, if it was not seen and you did come to the hospital when you did, if left alone would have grown bigger, and you would have not been able to get an operation to resolve the issue.

Is there any other questions the doctor asked? No I replied,she advise me to see my family doctor in the mean time. You will get a call from my secretary telling you the date and time of your operation.

After we left the doctors office and got home, I remained silent and disgusting walked into the bathroom looked into the mirror and cried for half an hour, then washed my face and went into the kitchen still not speaking, and made a cup of hot chocolate.

I sat and watch TV, trying to forget that what am about to face was my Goliath Cancer. After pondering what was steering me in my face, made a call to my doctor and asked for an appointment to see him the next day around 10:30 am.

After arriving for my appointment and entering the office waited for a while then the doctor called me into the room. Its always a pleasure talking to my family doctor had for over 35 years.

I told him about my operation for colon cancer and what he thought was my chance. He explained it in a way that understood. Lets say a horse in a race has 85% chance of winning and 15% chance of loosing how would you bet he asked? On the winning % i replied. There you go.

Your chances of beating the cancer is in your favour, so have no worries about it he said. Thank you I replied. He wished me all the best and left the office feeling very relieved. I drove home and relaxed for the rest of the day.

I spent a couple days relaxing at home, walking and waiting to hear from the doctors secretary about the date and time for my surgery. The only thing worrying me about the surgery was, would I have to walk around with a colostomy bag on my hip, or would I be normal as before my surgery.

It was the unforeseen or should I say the unknown which was putting the fear on my mind every time. Just was the thought about the outcome of the operation. That's when I prayed to God for his help, to ease my mind about the surgery.

Three days came and went as I waited patiently for the doctors call. It did not happened, not even on the fourth day of the week, although I was anxious to get my surgery over with showing patience is what was deeded by me, because nothing happens before it's time.

On the fifth day which was on the Friday of that week, after seeing my family doctor, I made a decision to sleep in a little longer than usual, just when the idea of sleeping a bit longer the phone rang. The other end of the receiver was the doctor's secretary.

Good morning she said, can I speak to calling my name? Yes, this is he. Your operation date is on Monday next at 8:00 am. You are to be there for 7:00 am to register and get ready for your operation. Your medication and instructions were forwarded to your pharmacy for pick up. Thanks you I replied and hung up.

After receiving the call, took a shower, got dressed and drove to the pharmacy for my medication. The pharmacist explained how it should be taken and wished me all the best. Returning home read the instructions again and relaxed for the day, and not thinking about anything.

On Saturday morning I made a huge breakfast because the next day which would be Sunday, would be a day of fasting and taking my medication in preparation for my surgery. At lunch time I made a good lunch, had chicken wings, potato salad and a smoothie.

In the evening I walked to the corner store, bought some drinks all of which were clear to drink on Sunday after drinking my prescribed medication. The more clear fluids you drind makes the flushing of your system much easier.

I remember not eating supper on Saturday, but drank a cup of tea, then went and lay down in bed pondering the outcome of my operation, knowing fully well it was out of my control. It bothered me a bit, knowing that having cancer was happening to me and not someone else.

It took me a while falling asleep on Saturday night. I remember tossing and turning in bed, not being able to fall asleep, walked into the kitchen, had a drink of water but only had a sip, instead of drinking the whole glass.

After returning to the bed room I laid on the bed and gradually fell asleep. The morning seems as though it was longer than usual, due to the dark drapes in the bedroom. It was about 9:00 am when I awoke from sleeping.

The hunger pangs and the grumbling started in my stomach, as though a pack of wolves had entered making it their home over night, knowing I could not feed my hunger.After eating all that good food on Saturday, today being Sunday it all have to be flushed out of my system beginning in three hour.

This was in preparation for my surgery Monday morning at 8:00 am something I was hesitant about but was necessary. It was time for me to begin taking my medication, but had to mix the powder portion with water, and it smell like vanilla cake before drinking the mixture.

In less than two hours, my stomach began rumbling like thunder, and the flood gate opened while sitting on the toilet bowl, and whatever I had eaten on Saturday came down as if it was shooting out from a water cannon into the toilet bowl.

The rumbling of my stomach and sitting on the toilet continued for most of the day, and part of the night until nothing was left inside my stomach. I had to drink clear fluids after taking the medication to make my system free from any leftover food. This process that I am going through would not do to my worst enemy.

It felt as though a plumber used his auger to clear the clog from my pipe system after all was completed, and nothing was left, all you heard was the sound like air brakes on a simi-truck when you pass gas or farted.

I tried sleeping early knowing in the morning (Monday) my surgery. After falling asleep, woke up very early, was driven to the hospital, and went directly to the oncology department, registered, and waited for all the procedures for my surgery was completed.

The doctor came and talked to me before my surgery, and explained what and how the procedure would be done, asking if I had questions, and said no but was scared and did not want anyone to know. She assured me that it would be fine because of the many operations she had done before mine.

As the time drew near for my operation, I was wheeled into the operation room on the bed that they had me lay on, and remember the doctor talking to me, a mask was placed over my nose, and knew nothing after that until waking up in the recovery room around 12:01 pm.

Two hours later I was wheeled into a semi-private room with another patient, and slept for about four hours. I remember after waking up the first thing that ran through my mind was feeling my side to see if they was a colostomy bag attached.

Luckily for me there was none, and thank God. In the front of me was a tray with two bowls one with jello and the other with pudding, and hanging a bag with clear fluid and a clear tube which was attached to a needle on the back of my hand, and drips flowing every couple seconds from the bag.

There was another clear tube with another bag that was hanging, and attached to that tube was a needle that was attached to my back, and remembered whatever liquid that was flowing through the tube had me itching, but had to wait until the doctor tells the nurse to remove it from my back.

I remember feeling my stomach area, and it felt as though they was a zipper over the bandages and yes there was what i found out later the doctor use staples instead of the usual sutures for this operation.

Making myself comfortable as possible, had no urge to use the washroom or even eat what was in the front of me. I was mostly interested in sleeping, not even talking, remaining quietly in my own thoughts, and praying silently everything would be good and back the way it was before my surgery.

I remember hearing a voice between sleep and wake calling my name, that walking would be good for me as much as possible to expel the air out of my body. To be truthful, I tried but was in so much pain, and went back to bed and lay down sleeping until the early hours of the morning when the nurse came to administer my medication and injection.

Today is day one after my surgery. I got up when the doctor called my name around 9:00 am and said good morning, asking me how was my night, and if they were anything that was making me uncomfortable, yes I said and told her about my itching problems.

The doctor removed the needle from my back, and it felt so good but encourage me to walk often as possible to relieve the pain the air is causing me. The doctor further explained to me what she had done during my surgery, and the amount of colon that was removed making sure she got all the cancerous polyps that was infectious out.

When I asked her how much colon she had removed her reply was about five feet. She sid the my colon was twisted inside and that I was one in a million that has so much. I was the forst person that she hd seen with that amount of colon.

After talking with me for twenty minutes she left to visit her other patients, that were on the same floor. I was again reminded to walk because of the built up air in my body walking would relieve the pain the more walking that is done.

It was difficult walking sometimes because of the excruciating pain that I was experiencing for the first time when ever walking around the wards, but had to make the effort to try and bear the pain. The most painful situation was when I had to cough or sneeze.

My experience with coughing or sneezing had to be improvised. After hugging a pillow close to my stomach every time when coughing or sneezing helped alleviate some of the pain. I did not eat or drink much, so; using the washroom was out of the question, because what was given to me to eat.

I was given soft foods to eat, all due to my surgery, and the doctor did not want me eating any solid foods at the time. For most of the day was spent walking and sleeping, did not watch TV or listen to the radio, but did some heavy thinking about what was next in the way of my recovery from Cancer.

I had just finished one of my courses at college before my surgery, but told none of my classmates about the surgery that was coming, but had registered for another course that was starting in January of 2004, but it was a wait and see scenario, how my recovery would turn out.

It is difficult sleeping tonight, due to the pain after my surgery, and it's worst because I cannot sleep on my stomach, or side only my back, sleeping on my side is difficult, since; I have to place pillows at my back propping me from rolling onto my stomach.

Although the room was quiet I found myself drifting asleep about 10:30 pm and dreaming just to find myself on a beach just laying on the sand under an umbrella enjoying the peaceful environment of the surroundings and the gentle breeze blowing as it cools your body down.

In between sleep and wake the nurse would stop by making sure everything was okay with the bag with the clear solution that it was dripping properly. I had the honour of wearing compress stockings, not my kind of dress code but it was necessary to prevent any blood clots from forming, although it felt uncomfortable at first I was getting accustom wearing it.

Today is day two Wednesday after my surgery, my morning began early around 4:30 am. I remember hearing a voice calling my name saying it's time for your injection, it was given every morning to help prevent blood clots in my legs.

After falling back to sleep it felt as though I was in a deep sleep, not being able to wake up, because of me being tired, and thought a voice was calling out my name once again but no one was around when I opened my eyes.

It was now time for breakfast just about 8:30 am half hour before the doctor makes her rounds visiting her patients. As the nurse pushed the breakfast cart with the food trays brought in my breakfast, of Quaker oats, apple juice, pudding and black tea. I went to the washroom brush my teeth and ate almost all of what was on the tray, leaving the pudding for later.

Have you ever eating hospital food? Then you will know, what I am talking about, especially lunch and dinner, at times being hungry was not even thought of, and was determined not to think that I was hungry. I wanted some real food with substance that taste like real food that was well seasoned.

The doctors voice was heard just before 8:55 am in the corridor and in five minutes she would be in my room for a visit. One thing for sure she was always on time her visiting time with me was always 9:00 am and today was no exception, she was right on time. She asked me how I was doing and if they were any bowel movements.

My reply to her was no, not yet, her words to me was if you do not have a bowel movement I cannot discharge you from the hospital. I will do my best, knowing for a fact it may never happen today.

I ate some of the leftovers and drank the liquid from the breakfast the day before, but could not eat the rice pudding it was not going down my throat no way no how. After the breakfast tray was cleared from in front of me I took a walk that was holding the bottle with the clear fluid.

After walking for a while I began feeling much better as the pain was beginning to ease that was causing my discomfort. There was not much to do but rest and sleep in order to gain my strength back. Today being the second day after my surgery I am hoping to have some visitors.

Yesterday was not a great day after my surgery, and did not want to see any visitors not even my family. Visiting hours at the hospital were from 4:00 – 8:00 pm. So; I had sometime to sleep and eat before visitors arrive ro see me along with my wife daughter and grandchildren.

Three of my friends came in together, looked at me and shook their heads, and said you look great. Thanks I replied considering what have gone through my feelings and out look was good. Although I was doing better it was no laughing matter because of the staples the doctor used to closed my wound, soon after about fivr minutes my wife, daughter and grandchildren walked into the room.

My grandchildren was kind of scared to come close to me, but stayed at a distance. It was not until I mention to them my illness was not contagious, they came closer. My daughter and grandchildren left half and hour after arriving, so did my friends, but before they left, gave them this advise please see that they get a colonoscopy soon.

Its best to make sure that your drainage system is running smooth, and was not being clogged by polyps. They agreed to do so when they can. My wife stayed a little longer and left a little before visitation time came to a close, promising she will be back again the following day.

I was getting a bit sleepy from the visits, and fell asleep soon after, then I was woken up ny the nurse, and had to take my medication. I could not get right back to sleep after my medication, and the gentleman that shared the room with me kept saying he was dying. He continued saying he was dying and wanted to talk with his family now which was impossible at the time, but fell back to sleep after the nurse came and speak to him.

It is Thursday day three after my surgery and I am slowly making progress with my recovery, along with my walking and my pains are now easing to a point where it can be tolerated. My morning routine started with a visit to the washroom to have a wipe down since it was impossible for a total wash.

After brushing my teeth and trying for a bowel movement which seems to be not forthcoming, no matter how hard I tried. The only good news that need sharing at this moment is my eating it has increased in the last day but everything else satys the same, lots of sleeping and walking with the odd visits from the nurse.

The doctor is always on time to visit with me she is here at 9:00 am and I can tell the time of her visits by her presence, cause it's the same every day without looking at the clock on the wall. Today's breakfast was good apple juice, Quaker oats, vanilla pudding and tea which was not bad.

I was still encourage by the doctor to continue walking often which would also help with my bowel movement. Am looking forward to the day when she can say to me you can go home where I can start eating some good homemade food.

Its not that the food here is bad its the taste just plain bland, and that is all the hospital food is, which is required by the doctor when there is a major surgery. As for the patient that wanted his family last night I have not heard any word from him, and his blind is closed. I cannot say for sure if he died during the nigh or not, or if he is still alive.

I can only do the best with what is given to me and the situation where am in at the present time. There is not much you can really do in the hospital except rest, relax and walk the floor and talk to other patients rather than the one that is in the same room with you if he speak your language.

In another couple hours will be lunch time, and I am only guessing today's menue for me would be soup, jello and apple juice cause its not advisable for me to have any solids yet. Although a menu card is on your food tray at every meal. You are limited to make a choice of food you would like, because what you want to eat is not available.

I am looking forward to visiting hours today, not sure if any more of my friends would be coming, but I do know my wife would be here but would be late because she works out of the city. All that I can say is I am being anxious to leave the hospital is an understatement.

But my condition does not warrant me leaving until I have a bowel movement and the orders comes from the doctor herself. At last there is some movement from the patient in the bed next to me. I heard a little sound and the nurse has just walked in to look after him.

Although I have not heard him asking for his family, except that one night ,when he was asking for them. Since I have been here no one came to visit him in the last couple days, may be he has no family that lives in the area.

Just as I was beginning to get hungry the food cart with the squeaky wheels came up the corridor and in came the nurse with my food tray, uncovering my food was chicken soup, apple juice, and jello. I was hoping for more than soup because I was very hungry and had some wolves to feed.

I took a walk after lunch and follow it with a long nap, got up just before visiting hours began, soon after a couple of my friends walked in and told them they could not make me laugh at the moment. My supper came in a couple minutes after and before my wife came.

She walked into the room gave me a kiss and we talked about her day and mine, and was glad my recovery had been progressing relatively good. My day was almost quiet as it could be until the patient sharing the room with me had visitors.

Their talking became very loud that it was not wise for me to be there, but he kept saying I am dying, and I want a big hamburger so; I left the room until it was quiet. I returned to the room after his visitors left, and went to bed soon after the nurse walked in to check on us.

She was making sure everything was okay. We are all all aware hospital food is what it is, and would stay that way unless changes are made. His moaning and grumbling kept me awake for sometime, and just when it became quiet saying to yourself I can sleep the moaning escapade started.

This time he was calling for the nurse, who finally came to his aid, and asking him to be quiet. At last peace and quiet returned and I can fall asleep, which was deprived to me in the stillness of the night. Just the occasional snoring was coming from the patient that shared the room nothing that would prevent me from sleeping until the morning.

It's 4:00am on day four after my surgery, and the nurse came into the room carrying a small tray with a needle and medication this is to prevent blood clots she said. I opened my eyes before she called my name, then she zap me with the needle on my stomach this tim instead of my leg.

I could not return to sleep, but laid on my bed thinking to myself it has been three days without having a bowel movement. And I don't think it will happen today. The feeling of having one was not there, but hope when it does my days at the hospital would be over.

In the past three days breakfast was served between 7:00 – 8:00 am. After that it was time for the doctors to make their rounds visiting their patients. My doctor was always on time 9:00 am and her bedside manners was superb always smiling and greeting me with a good morning.

The first thing she said to me after saying good morning was, did you have a bowel movement over night? No I said, she looked at me OK, guess you are here foe a while, only when you have that bowel movement you will be discharged.

She pent about ten minutes talking, and looked at my wound telling the nurse before leaving she can change the dressing. It's always a pleasure seeing the doctor before beginning my day. I look forward every morning to hear her voice in the corridor, before she enters my room.

This morning breakfast was good, Quaker oats, tea, toast with cream cheese. The only thing I did not like was the hospital gown you had to wear, with all your bare butt peeping out through the split at the back as though it was a broken window, while walking the corridor.

I had to make sure that I was holding the split together while walking, and also the bottle with the drip on the carrier. If you think you are a free spirit then you can let it fly wide open allowing everyone to take a look.

But my pride would not allow me to, I had to hold it for privacy. Today I told myself, walking longer steps and drinking lots of water should help me with my bowel movement it's something which I cannot wait for it to happen.

Not withstanding the pressure and the time you spend on the toilet, that's not happening at this moment. The gentleman in the room with me finally awoke, but was coughing a bit. I don't think he understands English very well, but it does no prevent him from saying what is bothering him.

I don't understand why his doctor has not visited him, since being in the same room. He had a couple family members visit him once, that I know off, and is not dying as he proclaim. Never have I seen him walk or got out of bed, but it's none of my business.

I have no idea what is wrong with him, or what type of surgery he had or any illness he is going through as he lay on the bed. Did walk a lot today before lunch and took a brief nap waking up in time to see the nurse walking into the room, with my lunch and medication.

After taking my medication I lift the cover off the lunch bowl, and once again it was soup with crackers, vanilla pudding, apple juice and tea. Now that lunch was over it's nap time before visitation begin later in the evening.

I am hoping not too many visitors would show up today, since being kept awake from the moaning and groaning from the patient that is sharing the room. Sleeping always came to me without any problems, and can fall asleep any time day or nightwithout any medication.

The only thing that would cause me to not fall asleep right away id distractions such as loud talking or loud music, and especially bright lights. Supper time is anytime between 4 – 5:30 pm, always around visiting time.

Some patients gets food brought in sometimes by family members, if and when they aske for it, other than that it's the food at the hospital. Today's supper were a couple potatoes mixed veggies, mash potatoes, apple juice, Jell-O and tapioca pudding. I made sure to eat all of it before any visitors came.

I am hoping by eating all that was served, will help me tomorrow with my bowel movement. It's a waiting period for it to happen, visitors began trickling in just after having finished eating. My daughter and grandchildren were the first to arrived.

Then two of my best friends after, leaving some room for others. It was standing room only for every one unless they wanted to sit on the bed. This visit was different for my grandchildren, they each came closer, without me asking them.

I had a great visit with them, they all wanted to know when would the doctor discharge me from the hospital, soon I said, and told them what was needed to be done before my discharge can happen.

Before leaving they came and gave me a small hug trying not to squeeze me too hard, and showed them wheremy incisionwas located. They said goodbye then left. My two friends stayed a little longer, but left after my wife walked into the room.

She did not stay long either because of the long day at work, not only that she had to get up early every morning to catch the train and to be on time at work. After she said her good night, and kissed me I fell asleep before 8:30 pm.

The night before was a tiring one because of my room mate who was moaning and groaning throughout the night. I was awaken by the night nurse around 10:00 pm she had to administered my medication, and to look after the bag with the drip, making sure everything was flowing properly.

Before falling back to sleep to sleep, they were some groaning coming from my room mate, and although we have never spoken, I felt sorry for him, because no visitors came to see him for a couple days.

I fell into a deep sleep after the groaning stopped, and was awaken by the nurse who came to administered my medication and injection for preventing blood clots around 5;30 am. After that stayed awake for the rest of the morning

It's Friday day five of my hospital stay after my surgery, and still have not gotten the urge to have a bowel movement. This is not a lack for not trying, it is simple not forthcoming. Although with all that was given to me was eaten that feeling was not even on the tip of my butt.

My breakfast today was two slices of toast, butter, tea, Quaker oats, and apple juice which I devoured like a vacuum cleaner, picking up the bits of left overs which fell on the floor, to say the least. Soon after my breakfast the good doctor walked into the room exactly at 9:00 am.

After saying good morning asked me a couple of questions one of which again was, If Ihad a bowel movement, and my answer was no, not today yet. It's still early in the day. She looked at my wound to see how it was healing, and said all is well.

She told me that the compression stocking can be remove, if I wanted which was certainly done without hesitation. It felt so good after wearing it for sometime, which was a breathe of fresh air for my legs making them feel comfortable once again.

I started my daily walk in the corridor after the doctor left after her visit, walked for half an hour and the urge to use the washroom was at the edge, arriving and sitting on the toilet seat, that very urge left me in an instant.

It was frustration to say the least, wow! I was very disappointed because i wanted it to happen so much, all because not having a bowel movement is all that is keeping me from being discharged from the hospital.

I had a nap after visiting the washroom, and slept until lunch time, when the nurse brought in my lunch, placing it on the table in front of me. The lunch meal was chicken soup, crackers, jello, and apple juice to say the least all tasted very bland.

After finished eating, had another walk, and entering the room, felt the urge to rush to the washroom, but not to have a bowel movement, but to vomit. My food was being rejected by my stomach. At this point my stomach felt empty, luckily for me I had a left overs of a pudding cup and juice from two days ago.

Which I did made use of, and had to wait until supper time to have something to eat. I called my wife and ask her to bring me something to eat, maybe a chicken burger and a drink, after her work. I was not looking forward to see any visitors today except my wife.

I know patience is a virtue, and I know that is all it takes, but five days and counting since my surgery and no bowel movements. My appetite was good and eating what was given to me, thinking by now, sitting on the toilet bowl they would be some activity with me having a bowel movement, it was not happening.

Laying on the bed all that was on my mind was having a bowel movement, so; I can getout of the hospital and start eating some rel food that is well seasoned and tasty. My thinking is, having a bowel movement is so that the doctor knows everything has been attached and is working the way it supposed to be.

I cannot see it any other way. Our supper was right on time and for supper was mash potatoes, peas and carrots, a small piece of chicken, apple juice and rice pudding for dessert. Eating everything except the rice pudding, I was patiently waiting on the chicken burger tat my wife was bringing, because my stomach was still feeling empty.

The clock on the wall showed the time as 6:30 pm and my wife had not shown up as yet, with my burger, but I know it was coming just that it was late and hated eating anything past 7:00 pm. Then I heard her voice in the corridor and she walked in kissed me and handed me what was requested with one of my favourite drink.

She stayed for an hour, ten left for home. It was dark outside because of the cloudy conditions. The sun was not visible today as previous days, soon after I was fast asleep, only to be waken by the nurse who was administering my medication and looking at the clear fluid making sure the drips were working properly.

Falling asleep tonight was easy, I had a full stomach. I awoke practically the dame time when around 4:30 am when the nurse came into the room to give me the injection to prevent blood clots.

Today is Saturday six days since my surgery and this morning I did not feel like doing anything much except laying in bed gazing up at the ceiling. I was not even thinking about breakfast, or the doctors visit, which I always looked forward to every morning since my surgery.

It was a busy day, some of the patients in other rooms on the same floor were being discharged later, and they were getting their things together. I wished them well as was walking by and went back to my room.

I hope today's breakfast would be much better than during the week an indeed it was. My breakfast was all good soft boiled eggs, toast, orange juice and tea still bland, but was much of an improvement from what I was eating before.

Just after I was finished eating the doctor walked into the room at the usual time. Asked me the same question she normally ask about bowel movement, and I replied no to her question. She looked at me called me by my name and smiled.

After taking a look at my wound she said everything was fine, and ask the nurse to put fresh bandage on it. I felt discouraged most of the patients on the same floor with me were on their way home at visiting hours.

I continued walking and drinking water often, and told myself today is the day my bowel movements will happened, don't know what time but will try and do everything possible for it to happen in a good way.

I was still walking around with the bag of clear fluid on the pole, only this time they was no pain even when laughing or sneezing, and felt that was progress in my healing. If only I can have a bowel movement, so; I would be able to go home like the other patients.

It will make me very happy indeed, and hopefully it will happen sooner than later. I kept looking at the time every ten minutes or so but it seems as though lunch would never arrived, soon after thinking that the food cart was being pushed, and my food was placed on the table in front of my bed.

I could not wait to see what lunch looked like and what a surprise, it was not soup but brown rice, chicken in a stew sauce, peas and carrots, orange juice along with a cup of jello for dessert. What I really hoped that after eating this food would help with my bowel movement journey.

It was just enough and filling for me after drinking the orange juice and having the jello. I took a walk and lay down for a short nap after. In the time of getting up my stomach started gurgling or boiling, and knew something was about to happen.

It was the moment I was waiting on for the last five days. I remember looking at the time as when entering the washroom, the clock on the wall said 3:00pm as my butt sat on the toilet seat. Yes, I said to myself home at last, and had a bowel movement which had eveded me for the last couple days.

It felt so good that I had a smile on my face, and all that I could think about was going home. The feeling felt as when you had sex and you made that ejection of vanilla cream tht oozed out of your man tube in a sweet squirt.

I was so happy, now and can answer the doctor's question if she ask me with a yes, after cleaning up walked out of the washroom with a smile on my face and all that was on my mind was going home the next day.

I was pleased with myself for accomplishing this feat which was evading me all this time, and was now looking forward to many more bowel movements. My thought were not having hospital food for supper, and wanted something from home.

So, I called my wife and asked her to bring me something to eat which she did. She brought me some fries, onion rings, and a cold drink. I was not expecting anymore visitor today, but two of my class mates showed up which was good and was gad to see them.

They left half an hour after arriving, and my wife stayed until visiting time was over. I told her about my bowel movement, and should be discharged tomorrow Sunday after seeing the doctor during her morning visit.

Tonight though could be my last night sleeping in the hospital, and all because of a simple bowel movement, as for my room mate I have not heard a sound from him or seen any visits from his doctor, it seems as though he is a forgotten patient.

I did have a peaceful sleep, but was also anxious when the morning comes, that my being discharged from the hospital once the doctor made her daily visits. Today is Sunday day seven of my hospital stay, and yes, had another bowel movement before breakfast.

Which puts me in a good position for getting discharged after breakfast. I waited for the time and the arrival of the doctor, and time seems to be going quite slowly. Just when I thought she was not going to show up at her usual time she walked into the room at 9:00am.

And right behind her was my wife who came in early making sure I was going to be discharged today. The doctor took another look at my wound and had the nurse replace it with a fresh bandage.

She asked me about my bowel movement, and told her I had one on Saturday afternoon, and the other this morning Sunday. She said to me, then you will be discharged, and would have to visit her office not at the hospital.

She gave me her office address where i need to see her. I smiled after she left to complete the paperwork for my discharge, began packing my clothes, and other items waiting on the words to leave and go home. My exit from the hospital was half an hour after talking to the doctor.

I was finally on my way home from the hospital, when I got home the first hospital the first thing was taking a sponge bath because taking a shower was out of the question, not until the visit to her office which was in a couple of days.

After having a sponge bath had something light to eat (tuna sandwich and orange juice) and had a good and peaceful nap for about three hours, and was waken up by the smell of food cooking in the kitchen.

I remained in bed very quietly, before entering thr living room to watch some TV programs, and have supper later. It was a lot different from the food at the hospital, but could not over eat, my inside needed time to properly healed before eating heavier food.

My days at home was spent very quietly resting, before the time came to visit the doctors office on the day that my appointment was given to me. I hope it would be good news, because some cancer patients, were saying they had undergo chemotherapy treatments.

I am hoping that it is not so in my case after my surgery. Its not so much as not doing the chemotherapy treatments but the condition it leaves you with, but the feeling and appearance it has on you in particular.

All I can say is everyone is different, and I may not have to undergo chemotherapy treatments at all, but it's not for me to decide. Today is Tuesday and my appointment with the doctor is at 9:00 am it's a close drive to her office. After getting there I checked in with her secretary, and waited until she called me to come into her office.

After entering her office and was greeted, sat down and she explained to me what she had done, and what was needed for me to do while I was recovering from my surgery. The thing she mentioned to me was that all the cancerous areas were removed from my colon.

That was in fact good news to my ears, but I would have to see my family doctor to have the staples removed where my incision were in another three days. She handed me the staple remover in a plastic bag which my family doctor would have to use to remove the staples on my incision.

Before leaving she told me to call her office if there is anything else I want to talk about. I left her office with a good feeling, knowing chemotherapy treatment was not in my recovery process, which was a good thing I think.

After returning home, had a cool drink of water, and went back to bed for a while. I made a call to my family doctor after getting up from my sleep,and asked for an appointment for Friday morning at 9:30 am and relaxed for the next couple days until my appointment time.

On the day of my doctor's appointment, I was a bit nervous, about how he was going to remove the staples. After he looked at it and gave him the staple remover it was a very simple procedure. It was all in my head that removing the staples were going to be painful.

I did feel a little pain but not as much. We chat for a couple minutes, then said good bye, left his office and went home. It was time to relax until my wife got home from work, did some packing of clothes to take to our cottage not to long a drive out of the city.

The days were starting to get cooler, and the leaves were starting to fall, and change their colors slowly, as the temperature declined daily in a time of transition. I enjoy spending time at the cottage because they were lots of things to do, gardening, cutting grass and my favorite fishing in the lake.

The only thing that i am not able to do at this time was going into the wate, and getting my stomach wet where my incision was, not until I think everything was ok to do so. It was only about an hours drive to the cottage.

I could not wait for my wife to get home. So we could be on our way to spend the weekend relaxing, and visiting a couple friends we made after buying the cottage. It was close to the time when she came home, and the keys could be heard at the front door.

By the way she jingle the keys I knew it was my wife, entering the apartment she relaxed for a bit then took a shower, packed some clothes, and we were off to the cottage for the weekend, promising not to do anything strenuous, but simple relax.

We stopped at the grocery store in the country to get a couple items for the weekend. I stayed in the car while she went inside to purchased the grocery items, since I could not lift any heavy items.

After a quick stop at the grocery store we arrived at the cottage, off load the clothes that we packed, the groceries, put them away, and had supper before relaxing and watching tv until it was time for bed.

Saturday morning came, and the sun was shinning through the window facing the lake. The wind was calm and the water on the lake was the calmest I have seen for a while in the last couple of weeks before my surgery.

After getting dressed I went for a short morning walk before breakfast. I returned to the smell of bacon, eggs, and toast sat down eat it all with a cup of hot chocolate to drink. My breakfast was delicious, not like the hospital food.

The breakfast dishes was washed and put away. We sat on the couch for a while before visiting our friends at their cottage, a couple cottages down from ours. It was okay walking but sitting was a bit uncomfortable because of the position I had to sit in.

I could not sit straight up in a chair, but more in a laying position. Saturday afternoon came so quickly after our visit and we were now preparing supper before watching TV helpimg us relax our stressful day.

It's a bit late in the evening, and as we looked out towards the lake the ripples on the water began as the wind became stronger. The temperature began to decreased making it much cooler, and it's a sign tonight will be colder than last night.

To take the chill out of the cottage we had to light the wood stove. This means getting some wood outside from the wood pile which were stacked along the fence. I got the wood stove lit, and waited a while for the room to warm up.

We continued watching TV and before going to bed. I had a hot cup of tea went to the washroom then off to bed. It's early Sunday morning, and the birds were chirping in the tree in the back yard that was on the lake side, with a bright sun and a gentle breeze blowing.

This Sunday I was not feeling to attend church, so; we took our time to prepare breakfast, and eat, and did any other food preparation we needed to get done before leaving the cottage, before we head home to the city.

It felt like a short weekend, that came so fast, but in a couple more weeks I will be staying at the cottage, during the weeks after feeling strong enough to be on my own. Then I can do all my cooking and lifting firewood for the wood burning stove to keep me warm and walking more.

It was time to pack the vehicle, to return to the city, before leaving we went to visit other friends in the area, had lunch at 2:00 pm and left around 3:30 pm to beat the traffic with cottagers returning to the city.

I spent the next two weeks resting and gaining strength, because I wanted to stay at the cottage the next time we go there. It also meant driving myself. It was agood two weeks for me, and found myself doing some walking, cooking, and baking some home made bread to take with us to the cottage.

The two weeks came, for me to drive myself to the cottage, and remain there for a while, a place that I enjoyed because of its tranquility and the peace it brought to me. Our drive to the cottage was not bad the traffic was good with less vehicles on the road.

I was going to remain there for a while. We stopped for groceries that would last me for the next two weeks before I return to the city. It was just getting dark when we arrived at the cottage.

As we approached the back of the cottage and look out towards the lake we could see a large ship with its lights on moving west slowly carrying iron ore towards a smelting plant that is located along the shore not to far from our cottage.

I got inside the cottage and started a fire to take whatever chill remained then went outside to help bring the groceries, and my clothes I would need for my days that would keep me here into the cottage.

It's going to be a great weekend, which started with having pizza and wings for supper with a cool drink while we watch a movie together, before calling it a night around 10:00 pm then we both went to bed until morning when the sun came up.

The nights were just starting to get a little cooler as the leaves on the tree began falling, giving way to the coming of the fall season, something I really don't really care much about, because after that cold weather begins bringing snow into the area.

After waking from sleep on Saturday morning, looking out towards the lake hoovering over the water was a thick mist. As the sun tried burning off the thick mist it would take a couple hours for it to happen.

I began preparing breakfast before my wife got up. We had turkey bacon, eggs, home fries, toast coffee for her and hot chocolate for myself. Sitting quietly for a bit, discussed our plans for the weekend.

Our plans for the weekend was cutting the grass, raking leaves, and making sure the plants were ready for the cold season that were ahead of us. It also meant firewood needed to be bought for the winter months. Although we had some that was left over from the previous winter we wanted to make sure we did not ran out of wood.

After breakfast and the dishes washed and put away, we relaxed for a few minutes before starting our weekend chores for the day and what was needed to be done. We did separate chores trying to accomplish as much as we could that Saturday morning.

We got a lot done and left the balance what little remained to be done on Sunday after church. It was time to fire up the BBQ, and we had some chicken, potato salad, and garden salad for supper.

After eating, sat on the deck watching the ducks swim by, envying them because I was not allowed into the water to do any fishing until getting the permission from the doctor to get into the water.

The dark skies came up quite suddenly, and the winds became much colder, forcing us to go inside. Just then the skies opened up and the rain began falling. You could hear the drops falling on the roof as though they were a marching band approaching.

Just as it started raining it suddenly stopped, and everything became quietly. It gave us time to clean up which was not much that we had to do. After we sat with a bowl of popcorn and watched a movie before going to bed around 9:30 pm.

It's Sunday morning, after a good night's sleep, we got ready for church which started at 8:3 am. We arrived at church early, enough to chat with friends before church commence, and talked about having brunch after church, so; we would not have to make lunch after we got home.

After church we did go for a brunch lunch got to the cottage about 12:05 pm we changed into some work clothes, and continued our weekend chores preparing the plants and the yard for the colder season. (winter)

A cooler breeze was beginning to blow and finished in time to prepare supper so my wife could head back home to the city. I was going to stay at the cottage to continue my recovery, while trying to gain strength that was lost due to my surgery.

After eating supper and my wife left for home, I just sat and watch TV for an hour had a warm shower, changed into my pajamas and laid in bed. Before falling asleep put another log into the wood stove to keep the inside warm during the night until next morning.

For the next couple of days I would be by myself, and making sure to keep busy walking and visiting with friends and doing the odd cleaning around the yard, and taking lots of naps during the day.

I made sure that it was necessary for me to eat at the same time every day and sleep for about eight hours, only getting up in the morning, when the urge of hunger was coming on. The days flew by, and so was the months, as the colder weather rear its ugly head.

We were prepare to face the winter whatever it threw at us, winds or heavy snow, which was common with living close to the lake. I did not hear from the doctor who did my surgery, but from what she said was she had gotten all of the cancer in my colon taken out. They should be no need for me to have chemotherapy treatments.

It was the last Sunday in October 2003, and was surprise that evening when I got a call from the Cancer Hospital telling me that my appointment with them was at 9:am on Monday morning, that's tomorrow I said, yes it is was the reply.

I was not expecting to have any chemotherapy treatments I said, but will be there. She gave me all the information needed that I need to get done before getting my first treatment on Monday morning.

My wife tool Monday off from work, to take me to the Cancer Hospital, but before visiting the doctor who was in charge of the chemotherapy treatments I had to get an x-ray first and blood text second and the third thing was to get weighed and measure my height.

After getting through all the necessary tests, made my way to see the doctor carrying my x-ray and all the information about myself. I handed him the information, and he explained everything that was going to happen to me today.

I sat in the waiting room until my name was called, walked into the room where my chemotherapy treatments were going to happen. After sitting in the chair I was given a warm blanket to cover myself.

My first day of thirty sessions of chemotherapy was about to begin. The nurse who was administering the treatment came up to me and introduce herself. She gave me a cup of ice and told me to place some between my gum and teeth in front of my mouth.

I did not ask any questions, but did what she said, she cleaned the area on the back of my hand where she was going to place the needle shaped like a butterfly. I watched her placed the medication through a tube that was connected to the needle.

I felt a cold sensation flowing through my veins, on the back of my hand, and tasting something that I had never tasted before, but she continued telling me to put the ice between my gum and teeth.

My chemotherapy session lasted twenty minutes. I felt fine walking away but had to return the next day four day for treatments. My stomach began growling because of the time I had to be at the cancer clinic time was not of the essence for an early breakfast.

On the way back to the cottage, we stopped at a restaurant to have a quick breakfast, before returning. After sitting at the table and ordering our breakfast of eggs, turkey bacon, home fries ,toast, orange juice and tea.

We had to wait for at least ten minutes before it was served, but it was worth the wait. It looked very delicious, and yes it was. I began eating after putting some catchup on my home fries, and began eating everything tasted great.

What I remember half way through my breakfast was feeling a bit nauseated, and before reaching the washroom vomiting half of my breakfast on the floor in the hallway, between the dining room and the washroom.

My wife had to explained to the waitress what had cause me to vomit, and they were understanding about the whole incident. I returned after making sure everything was okay, before continuing to eat and finish my breakfast.

It was a good thing I was not driving, and it did not happen in the vehicle. After leavingthr restaurant and getting to the cottage, changed into more comfortable clothes and went to bed for about five hours. I got up to use the washroom, and went back to bed until the next morning to repeat another rounds of chemotherapy again.

Today is Tuesday my second day of chemotherapy treatment, and had to drive myself to the cancer clinic, because my wife had to work. I had to go through the same procedure this time the doctor did not require any x-ray.

Before my treatment, I explained to the nurse what had happened yesterday after my treatment. She was so kind to tell me the doctor should have told me about getting nauseated, and gave you a prescription for pills to control it. She gave me one and after my session went to the pharmacy at the hospital and got those pills for the nauseating which helped quite a lot.

I returned to the cottage after my chemotherapy treatment, after changing my clothes had toast and hot chocolate then went directly to my room laid on the bed and slept for about six hours, had something light to eat and went back to sleep.

Today is Wednesday it's day three of my chemotherapy treatment. I got up early and left early in time to start the process all over again, another two days before I get a rest to recuperate from my first week of treatments.

I was reminded that my chemotherapy treatments would be thirty sessions all together, of one week of treatments and three weeks off, with another two days left of my first week ending on Friday.

I would not have to return until three weeks after Friday giving me time to rest and take it easy in which time the cancer clinic will call and let me know my next appointment times. It did not feel so bad this first couple days but do not know how the other treatment would affect me.

Today is Friday my last chemotherapy treatment for the week, and thank God I have made it through with out getting nauseated as my first day treatment. I slept for four hours after returning to the cottage, and got up after a restful nap.

It's late Friday evening when my wife arrived at the cottage for the weekend. She entered the cottage and we chat for a bit, asking me ,how are you feeling? And told her how the chemotherapy treatment was making me feel.

My first week of chemotherapy was not that good, but I had no choice in the matter. It felt bad on the first day after vomiting and feeling nauseated at times. After it took three days of chemotherapy where my body system was beginning to accept the medication.

My first week is over and I am now on a three weeks resting period before having the next five days straight treatments again. In the meantime I have to rest on daily, while awaiting the next set of treatments.

Today is Saturday morning the sun is up and the reflection on the lake was like sparkles on the water. At breakfast whole eating my toast for the first time I could not taste the toast because it was bland, but continued eating due to hunger.

It's the first time in my life where that I had lost one of my senses, my sense of taste. There was only one thing that I could think of at that moment, but the chemotherapy medication for this lost.

What else could happen? It was a wait and see, how it would turn out as my treatments goes. I felt good, we went for a walk after breakfast and visit some friends, because it was not capable for me to do during the week of my chemotherapy treatments.

My time was mostly spent sleeping after my first week of treatments, and also eating trying to regain some strength what was lost from the chemotherapy treatments. For the rest of that month my breakfast was simple toast with butter and Quaker oats.

For lunch it was chicken soup with whole wheat crackers and a cold drink of cranberry juice. My supper was baked chicken with veggies with one of my favourite drinks, either malt or peanut butter, banana and frozen yogourt smoothie.

I visited my friends at their cottage every morning around 10:00 am after my breakfast the weeks I am off from chemotherapy treatments, for about two hours. After visiting returned by 12:01 pm to have my lunch and sleep for a couple hours.

Always getting up in time to prepare my supper, it was either chicken soup, or stew chicken with rice, beans and sweet potatoes. It was not always the same food each day. I made sure of eating certain foods that was good for me to gain my strength.

Some days was colder than others because it was during the winter months. I had to go through my treatments, and although it was cold my walking had not stopped, exercising and bringing firewood inside to keep the cottage warm enough from feeling cold.

After two months of Chemotherapy and feeling the effects of the medication that has place your whole body in an uneasy state, not knowing what the next treatment would bring to affect your health it was my commitment to continue with school, in order to graduate with my classmates.

Although attending classes were out of the question, my school work along with the notes and assignments were faxed to my wife by one of my classmates. All the notes and assignments was given time for me to hand them in after my wife brought them on a Friday evening.

I remember having supper on a Saturday evening after one of my chemotherapy treatments, and just after having the last bite of chicken it did not feel right and had to make a dash to the washroom and vomit everything I had eaten for supper.

After that episode had a hot cup of hot chocolate change into my pyjamas and went to bed. My wife left me and went for a visit to our friends, returning a couple hours after. It felt that the medicine that I was getting from the chemotherapy treatments were doing harm to my body but did not know what it was doing.

The teacher at college gave me enough time for my assignments and could call if I was not feeling well for an extension. All my treatments, except for the first two months were during SARS, and no one but the patients or those having an appointment were allowed into the hospital or cancer clinic at the time.

I was fortunate enough to continue my studies and still go through with my treatments. All during the time I was hoping that one day it was possible to surprise my classmates, before the term ends.

The hardest thing for me was driving myself to these chemotherapy treatments, because of not knowing how I will feel after a treatment. I had to make sure that everything was okay for me to drive back to the cottage.

They were times I wish chemotherapy was not part of my treatments for cancer, because it left me with so much deficiencies, like my fingernails changing color, becoming brittle and always splitting down the middle of my nails.

I don't know how long these deficiencies would last but if it does there are no other choices. There are still another three months left in my chemotherapy treatments, and my body is finding it hard at times to adjust after the second month.

In the forth month of the second day I remember it was going to be just another day of chemotherapy. My regular nurse that administered my treatment was off that day. I had another nurse attending to me.

She did everything right until the chemotherapy medicine began flowing, instead of it going throw my vein it was causing the back of my hand to swell. Whatever she did was not right and the cold sensation I felt and the feeling as though my hand were on fire causing me to yell! Take the needle out.

I told her to get someone else to administered the chemotherapy medicine. I felt bad for her but if it had done right the first time my yelling at her would not have happened. After my treatment I found her and apologized.

The six months of going through chemotherapy treatments was not easy for me. It has now began to take a severe effect on me, as it went along, sometimes I found myself feeling sleepy or just plain exhausted.

My school work was not getting done on time, because of how I was feeling during the day. I was given time to complete it as quickly as I can, and fax it to the teacher for which the support he gave me.

I made the extra effort to do the assignments and to complete them on the weekends. They were times I could not concentrate on my school work and just gave up and went to bed, because it was difficult. The way the chemotherapy treatment had an effect on me.

The idea of me thinking it was possible to do chemotherapy treatments and school work was a stupid idea, all entirely. It was something I had to prove to myself that in the situation graduating with my classmates was possible.

After completing my thirty bouts of chemotherapy treatments, and feeling stronger. I gave myself another three weeks at home, and surprise my classmates showing up at school for a class. They were all happy to see me when I walked into the classroom unannounced.

My classmates wanted to know how I was doing, and got a get-well card signed by everyone. It proved to me that i was really missed at school and among my peers. I eventually continued attending school and completed the term.

I graduated with my classmates thanks to one of the students that made it possible and the teacher for giving me the allotted time to complete my assignments. It was hard work and was proud of myself for putting the effort into making it happen.

Three weeks after graduating, and completing my chemotherapy treatments, my sense of taste was not back. I remember having a piece of toast with with butter, and I could not taste anything it tasted bland, and thought I have lost my taste for good.

My nails were still discolored, brittle, splitting, and breaking more often thaan before having chemotherapy treatments. I felt hopeless in a way that there was nothing that could be dome for me at that moment.

I was spending more time at our friends during the week because my wife was only at the cottage on weekends. Being by myself I was also walking for longer periods in the mornings after breakfast. My toast still tasted bland with either jam or cheese.

I did not know, how long my sense of taste would last? It did not stop me from enjoying whatever I cooked. My guess is it's one of the sensation you loose when you have cancer and have to do chemotherapy treatments.

What I can remember was, three months after chemotherapy, and not being able to taste any toast. But one morning while having a cup of hot chocolate, and toast with butter and cheese, biting into the toast I could taste the toast after a long time.

My sense of taste was back to normal. The taste of toast came back just as it left, and I could eventually enjoy my food once again. It was something I did not take for granted, which is very important to know, when you have cancer, and have to go through chemotherapy treatments.

The chance of not only loosing one of your senses like taste is there. I know because of the experience of having chemotherapy treatments cause me to loose my sense of taste it depends on how strong the medication is for your chemotherapy.

The chances of loosing you hair is another thing that is a possibility, luckily for me I had no hair to lose because of being bald head. I returned to work after all my chemotherapy treatments and school were completed.

My return to work was on limited days and the amount of hours allowed at the time was four hours a day only working three days a week. could work until. The only way that it was possible for me to work a full eight hours day was if I felt stong enough and with my doctors permission.

I worked two months part-time and was back to my normal hours working days for the next year without any days feeling sick. One day I got a call from the doctor telling me that i am due for another colonoscopy.

I made an appointment to see her at her office, and she explained that it was compulsory to have a colonoscopy every year, for the next five years, to make sure everything was going ok. She gave me a date and time for the colonoscopy procedure.

The list of the medication I need to take a dfay before the procedure which was nothing that was not done before. I had colonoscopies done every year for the first five years (2003 – 2005) then every other year for five years.

My colonoscopies are done now every three years the last one was done just around 2020 and I am due now in 2024. all this is to make sure that polyps was not forming as a cancer cell that may need surgery again.

I keep telling my friends, family, co-workers and anyone who would listen to me that they should have a colonoscopy test done, because the stool test that is given out is not telling or giving you a true sense of security that you do no have cancer of the colon.

The stool test cannot tell you if you have polyps, or if they are cancerous or not. The only thing it tells is if you have blood in your stood, and it can or maybe too late for you, if blood is seen on the stool sample test.

I know men are very reluctant to see a doctor they will tell you they are fine when really they are not. I have lost my best friend to leukemia cancer, and the other to throat cancer a year apart all because they did not want to go and see a doctor.

It is very important for you as a man or woman after the age of forty-five years to get a colonoscopy done today. You should ask your doctor about it. If you are denied, get a second opinion. I was luck enough to feel a pain on the inside of my shoulder. They were no signs of me having any symptoms of cancer that I knew off.

I don't want you getting me wrong but am glad to have had cancer at that time, than later in my life. Then I may have lost the will to live. It is something I can say now because looking back all those twenty plus years, my appreciation is that being alive and knowing not too many people live after having colon cancer.

We all know trhat colon cancer goes by another name of colorectal cancer. I am not here to tell you how to live your life, but here to give you the details of my journey with cancer and chemotherapy treatments.

The Goliath that I had to face head on, and came out a winner. I am not here to tell you the signs of your symptoms, my sign was a simple pain that took me to the hospital, and things mushroom from there. I was lucky enough that they did lots of different test plus a biopsy and found cancer on my colon.

You can research the symptoms of colon cancer, or refuse to do so it's your choice. If you are the kind of person like me, who heeds the advice of afriends who has gone through the experience of having colon cancer, you will take his warning.

The fact is colon cancer or for that matter have no age limit. Its best to have a colonoscopy test done if it runs in the family. If the foods you are eating are red meat and heavy processed you need to take a look at your diet and cut back on the amount you are consuming.

These foods are contributors of colon cancer. The truth is any kind of cancer can be beaten if you are in-tuned with your body. Any thing you find that is not normal with you see your family doctor do not wait for the symptoms to persist longer when it is unbearable.

Any kind of pain, bloating, weight loss, for no reason, constipation, and anything you are aware of please see your doctor and ask for that colonoscopy procedure. Its your health and it is important to you.

I was fortunate to have a great doctor with a great bedside manners, who was punctual every day of my hospital stay. She was always on time, and did not have to look at the clock to see what time it was the minute she walked into the room.

My cancer surgery and chemotherapy treatments were done at two different hospitals in the city of Hamilton in Ontario Canada, it's the home of the four best, my surgery was done at one the best St. Joseph.

Its has been twenty- one years since I was diagnosed with colon cancer, and gone through chemotherapy treatments. Just having survive it, was all due to my diligence, and always looking after my health.

I will mentioned once again, my family doctor had me on a diet, no eating of red meat or any kind of process foods, but eating lots of food with fibre, which would help in lowering bowel cancer. In the end its not what I say to you.

It all comes down to what you have read, the advice you take and the choices you choose to make, with the changes to your diet and exercise. Every decision you make in life would affect you, if it's a bad choice.

Whether or not you choose to change the way you view what you eat, or do it's up to you as an individual. The time to get a colonoscopy is not yesterday, tomorrow but today. So; make that call to your doctor.

Please make sure you get a referral to have a colonoscopy done and that everything is okay with you. With it out of the way you are good for another year until you get another colonoscopy test.

I had a Goliath standing in my way which I had to face. And am not saying it was not fearful, because it was, but facing it head on with help from my friends and family, I was ready to do battle no matter what situation laid ahead of me.

In the end I came out a winner leaving all the fears that was in the beginning of my journey. I also did a lot of praying while waiting, and before the day ofmy surgery. It's my faith along with my beliefs in Jesus that I was able to overcome my Goliath.

We all have Goliath's in our lives, staring us to our faces. When we look into the mirror I don't know what each of you who are reading my journey is facing. One thing i know is we can overcome whatever it is, by having a strong faith and believing it can be won.

Its strange when we think about it. The only time most of us pray is when we are facing a crisis, illness or dying within the family. We never think that our prayers are always answered, but not in the time you and I need it, which is right away, this very instant.

We all fear what we cannot see, and cannot control, but people who has a deep christian faith, do not let fear which is another Goliath have a strong hold on them. If you put your trust in Jesus and believe that He is the healer, and the great physician you are in good hands.

For my inner system to work the way it should, avoiding any more polyps my diet had to modified. I had to eat more fiber, vegetables, fish and chicken instead of red meat(beef) and any meats that was heavily processed.

I must say that it's a blessing to have survive colon cancer, and writing about it is my way of letting you the readers of this book what my perplexing situationwas. It's all about the journey that I had to take for me to get over this deadly disease called colon cancer.

If it was not diagnoses or left untreated would have been fatal. Do not take your health as a joke? It's not something to play as a game. If at any time you are not feeling well, the way you normally do, check in with your doctor.

We are well aware in this era, what cancer of any kind can do if not caught early to your health. If you think you are invincible then play as it was a game and that you have nine lives as a cat. If you are thinking as a human being where death is inevitable look after your health.

You do not have to prove to anyone that you are healthy if you are sick. Do not pretend to your friends? The only one you are really hurting is yourself, family and friends. I am not a doctor, just some person that had colon cancer.

I am just one of many that know the journey my cancer took me on. It is not something I would wish on anyone. The only way to avoid getting colon cancer is to try eating healthy, frequent check-up with your family doctor not a walk-in clinic.

The foods we eat and know that are contributors to this disease, must be avoided if possible. If you have the ability to cook do so, instead of eating out at the fast food burger joints. Eating lots of fibrous foods less red meat, and heavily processed food can help reduce your chances of colon cancer.

Like I said before. You have to know your body and your inner system how your plumbing system works. If your gut is telling you something is not right listen to what's its telling you, do not take chances with the slightest pain.

I was one who took my pain seriously enough to walk to the hospital, and had a series of tests. It turned out that cancer was causing my pain in my inner shoulder. During my chemotherapy treatments they were people that had to wear the colostomy bag.

It is not for me to judge anyone as to why they had to wear the colostomy bag. They each had this answer, their doctor wanted them to wear it because another surgery was going to be performed after their chemotherapy treatments to do a reattachment. That in itself was another distraction in this whole situation having colon cancer

The way I see it things could have been worst, the possibility not being alive and being alive and live through the ordeal that you can relate to or you could have been sent home to spend your days waiting to die. The choice they made and the faith they have in their doctors says it all.

What isneeded on our part to do when we go to the washroom is to be aware of whet our poo looks like. The more frequently we have a bowel movement that looks like diarrhea, or thin like a pencil it should raise a red flag.

This sign shows that you may already have cancer forming from polyps, that are in the early stage of cancer. The earlier we notice any sign it's time to see your doctor, insisting that you would like to get a colonoscopy test done.

Some of the signs that we need to be aware of are pain in your stomach and fatigue which could be give away signs of undiagnosed cancer. By checking yourself after using the toilet is a way of looking at your poo, for any signs of blood.If there is it's time to have a serious tlk with your doctor.

Are there signs that you need to be aware of; yes, here are some of the signs you need to be aware of changes in your poo, diarrhea or constipation you never had before. All these could be early warnings signs of colon cancer

If you go to the washroom often, and your poo is blood red or black when you see blood after you wipe, it's a sure sign that you are indeed have colon cancer. There is no need to be scared it good that you see it now that much later.

There are other other signs that have to be paid close attention to,the feeling that you need to poo although you had just had a bowel movement, any pain that you may feel in your stomach or any lump that you may have felt or detected,that you have seen while standing in front of a mirror.

Other signs that you have to be aware of is bloating and loosing weight for no reason. You need to take action right away, ask yourself the question why am I having these signs when I am eating healthy? Is there something wrong with what in my food.

Do not wait and say that it will go away as fast as it came. It might be too late. The fact that you have never seen or had these signs before is a clear indication something is definitely wrong with my inner system.

Sometimes these signs could be also caused by some other health conditions. It does not mean that colon cancer is already present. What is it telling you is its a warning sign for you to see your doctor.

Like I said before if cancer is detected early, it can be treated before it becomes to a stage where there is no hope, but to wait for your life to end. The choice we make with the knowledge we have about cancer is the best way I know.

Another sign that you have to be familiar with and be aware of is fatigue or feeling tired for no reason.Colon cancer can cause anemia making you feel tired, breathless and also can cause headaches.

There are no reason for you to be scared, but it's a wake-up call that you take cancer seriously and your health. Looking after yourself and doing the right things you can be sure to avoid having colon cancer.

I am only a messenger like John the Baptist, just letting you know that what you have to be aware of the journey you would have to endure if and when your turn come that you do have colon cancer. The things that you may have to lose during your chemotherapy treatments.

There are times I think about my cancer although it's in remission, that it can return. Having gone through with chemotherapy does not men it cannot. The only way it may return is not eating the right kind of foods, but returning to the way I ate before my cancer.

During my chemotherapy, one of the things I had to do was staying away from anyone that had a cold, flu, or any illness, because my immune system was very much depending on me staying healthy to get through the treatments.

Some of the ways I kept my immune system strong as possible during my chemotherapy treatments were: sleeping, eating, walking, being stress free, and not getting sick. You have to understand that any kind of treatment you are doing whether it's chemotherapy or radiation they can cause your immune system to get low.

Lets take a look at the ways these five things can help your immune system stay strong .

Sleeping:Getting more than 8 hours of sleep. Going to bed at the same time if possible every night and waking up. Always going to bed not hungry but feeling satisfied. Sleeping with your bedroom dark, cool and quiet.

Eating:Know what foods to avoid. Do not eat foods that says may help you boost your immune system. Eating healthy foods that is good for your immune system. Quaker oats, nuts, well cooked foods like poultry.

Moving:I found the more walking that was done the better. If you think you are not capable it's ok, but do whatever you can. Some of the causes that you may notbe able to walk for any length of time is; if you are extremely fatigue, low red blood cells which can make you (anemic),poor muscle, not being strong in your legs or low white blood cell count.

Managing Stress: One of the ways that helped me was listing to classical music, while resting and relaxing on my bed or lying on the couch, and thinking about nothing but the peaceful mood and way the music mesmerized you.

Illness: Anything that can give you and adverse reaction, bad food, food preparation, germs, not cooking poultry to the right temperature not washing fruits and veggies properly, or not rinsing salads that are in packages.

I have never given any thought to the food that I ate during my chemotherapy treatments. Eating what was cooked and avoiding red meats and processed foods. What ever was not tasting right for me was avoided.

No one ever told me that eating certain foods was not good or not to eat. But knowing what may cause an adverse effect on you after eating them was a clear indication that you should stay away from if it will cause any discomfort.

There are foods that you can eat, if you think you can handle them without causing you any side effects. What we eat during treatments can cause some ups and downs with our apatite and body weight.

It's very important to pay attention to any diet you may choose. The one thing that is certain is maintaining a healthy weight during chemotherapy or radiation treatments. We all know that eating healthy can promote a positive outlook in our lives.

Eating healthy helps in so many ways during and after chemotherapy or radiation treatments like .

. Reducing side effects.

. Giving us more energy.

. Helps us to tome our muscles.

. Helps to maintain our immunity system.

. Decreases inflammation.

There are foods that we can all eat and should during treatments that can help us stay healthy. Foods that are rich in.

Proteins: For instance Veggies, beans, nuts and seed. Eating animal proteins that are lean meat (not red meat) chicken or fish.

Healthy Fats: Avocado, olive oil, walnuts, are all good, and they helps with inflammation while improving cardiovascular health.

Healthy Carbs: Foods that have little or no processing, like whole wheat, beans, and oats which can help maintain good bacteria in the gut.

As long as you maintain a good and healthy diet when you are eating food that are good choices. You should not have any problems. The choice of foods you choose to eat in your diet plans are all up to you.

I wished that they was a dietitian while doing my treatments but unfortunately for me they was none available, so; all my food was based on trial and errors to see what my stomach could handle.

My foods were simple I ate only what I liked and did not go beyond trying anything new, that would make it difficult for me. I approach food with caution and what my stomach could handle at times it was fearful to eat because some foods sent me to the toilet less than half hour after eating.

As I look back on my journey with cancer and chemotherapy treatments, it never occur to me that my pain on the inside of my collar bone area was the sign that saved my life. If the pain was eased with the concoction I was drinking who knows where and how my life would be like today.

It is imperative that you as an individual that you know the family medical history. I did not realized that once cancer is in your family, you are most likely to be a canidate. That is why its important to know the facts about cancer.

I remember my aunt on my mothers side of the family having stomach cancer. She was told it could be an ulcer but in fact it turned out to be stomach cancer but it was inoperable. She was admitted to the hospital and remember driving from Canada to New York to visit her, while she was in the hospital.

When I entered the room she was in and she heard my voice she knew it was me. I gave her a soft hug and talked for a while before returning to Canada. Three days later she died and had to return to New York for her funeral two days after her death. It was a sad moment for me.

My best friend that I grew up with during childhood also died. He was sick for a while and the doctors did not know what was causing his illness. He was hospitalized for a couple days and sent home. Soon after within a day he was back in the hospital getting worst.

It was not until his daughter who is a nurse in England came down to see him that she saw the signs that she knew and told the doctors her father Leukemia. He died a couple days after, it was another sad day in my life.

Cancer also was also close to me a couple years after I was diagnose with my colon cancer my younger brother had cancer and was treated using radiation. He is better know but it is now part of our family history.

Cancer is a disease that can put you on a collision course with death. Your health is very important, and what you eat can be detrimental. I urge you who are reading what I had to go through on my journey look after yourself health-wise, and be good to yourself.

I have another colonoscopy test coming up soon after three years but I already know that there are some polyps that needs to be taken care of. It was not possible to have it done before due to Covid-19 but it is schedule within the month of July 2024. Its something that must be done if I have to stay as healthy and not allow the cancer to return.

The day for my colonoscopy test have arrived and today is Monday. I am starting my medication preparation that is needed for my test tomorrow Tuesday. Today Monday it will be a constant journey to the toilet after taking the medication for a total clean out.

It won't be easy starting at noon, until the end that I can see clear fluid exiting the toilet bowl and all the gas I will be passing is only air. My night sleep was peaceful with out using the toilet for any emergencies.

Today is Tuesday, and was driven to the hospital for that all invasive test called a colonoscopy, after registering was given two gowns to put on and then a needle was placed into my vein which would allow the medicine would be placed to put me to sleep for the procedure to be carried out.

I was wheeled into the room where the procedure would be carried out and after signing the consent form was given the dose that put me to sleep. After my recovery and was able to walk without wobbling was sent home. It was a chance for me to sleep for the rest ofvthe evening.

I only had something to eat after waking from sleep and went straight back to bed, sleeping through until next morning. My breakfast was a bowl of cereal and tea, relaxed until it was time for me to returned where I live in another city away from my daughter.

For the next two days I spent resting and watching a movie until it was time for me to continue my normal routine. It is something that I must say in spite of having a colonoscopy they were other things the doctor saw, and now have to change my diet once gain this time eating lots more fibre. I am good for another three years before another colonoscopy test.

Do not think cancer only happens to older adults. There is a rise where people under the age of 50 who are now in the majority situation of getting cancer. It is now become a concern concern, in the rapid rise of colon cancer with young adults, and this form of cancer needs to be addressed by the medical authorities.

The fact that we are now seeing a rise in more young adults, being affected with colon cancer is, because of their life style, and the foods they are consuming. The foods that are heavily contaminated with preservatives, and processed with lots of additives are the culprit for the onset of young adults being affected with cancer.

Most young adults think they are invincible. They need to think about it and change what they are consuming daily. We all tend to ignore any signs that are related to this disease, and pass it off a joke, when it should be taken seriously, and not regard the feeling that you are having.

You may think cancer would never touch you, think again. I have said it, that my sign for finding out that I had cancer is totally different to yours and was glad that I paid attention to my feelings.

The crucial signs for detecting cancer at it's early stages are:

1. Blood in your Stool

It's a sign that somethings are not right, and the colour of your stool can have the appearance of bright red blood or dark black tar like stool which are tell tales signs that something is wrong with your digestive system.

At this point a consultation with your family doctor, insisting that you need a colonoscopy should be your choice to clear the air if they are any doubt in your mind. This is not to be taken lightly.

2. Any type of Constipation

Any change to your bowel movements, recent changes can be a sign of colon cancer. It's not always the case, but can be cause by what you consume. If it occurs with pain in your abdomen, and blood in your stool, you should visit the doctor and seek advice.

3. Anemia

It's a deficiency of the red blood cells, a symptom that is a signal of colon cancer when it cannot be explained. It is caused by chronic blood loss from cancer tumor, which is not visible. Blood work along with imaging is helpful in this case to determine if colon cancer is a factor.

4. Weight Loss

If for no reason, you suddenly start loosing weight it should be a red flag. You may have some kind of cancer, especially if you have not changed your diet or exercise habits. It is known that cancer cells can alter the body metabolism, when it comes to loosing weight if we are eating normally.

Tumor in the colon may cause one to feel full quickly or lose theie appetite, which can be a contributing factor to their weight loss.

5. Abdominal Pain

Constant pain that would not go away is a common symptom of colon cancer, it can range from a mild discomfort to a severe cramp, and can be associated with our digestive issues. This pain is cause by the obstruction of a tumor, or the cancer may have already spread to other tissues nearby.

Young adults, experiencing such pain woth other signs mentioned should heed the warning, no matter how minor it is. They should seek medical advice from they family doctor to get an early diagnosis about the cause.

If we all eat healthy, and see what is written about what causes cancer you will find that it boils down to the high amount of preservatives and processes foods we consumes daily. Do not be another statistic of cancer.

Don't miss out!

Visit the website below and you can sign up to receive emails whenever Adrian Hamilton publishes a new book. There's no charge and no obligation.

https://books2read.com/r/B-A-PFIR-ERHTE

BOOKS 2 READ

Connecting independent readers to independent writers.

Also by Adrian Hamilton

Confusing Mind Confusing Time
Thoughts Expressions and Feelings " The Reality of Being"
LOVE LETTER'S FROM DISTANT LOVER's
Victor and Annabella
Faith and I
Death by fire
Death by fire
Dismembered
My Goliath

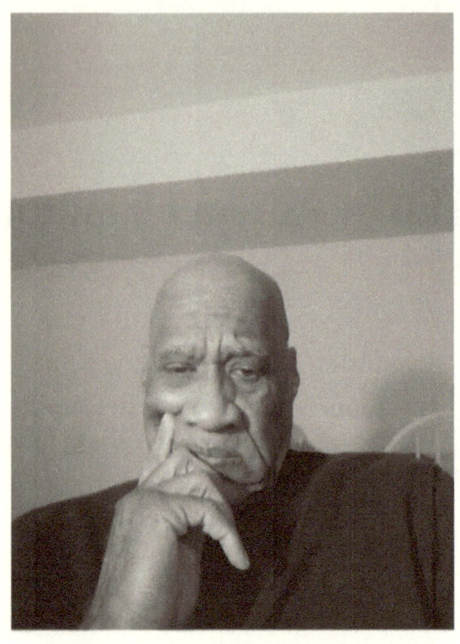

About the Author

Father of two children, with three grandchildren, and a greatgrandson comes from a family consisting of three boys and four sisters.He interest are fishing, hiking,and walking. He resides in the City of Mississauga, Ontario Canada.